KETO DIET COMPLETE BEGINNERS GUIDE

THE SIMPLEST, NATURAL, THERAPEUTIC AND PROVEN WAY TO LOSE WEIGHT AND IMPROVE YOUR HEALTH AND YOUR GENERAL WELLBEING

DR. KRIS GUNNARS

TABLE OF CONTENT

INTRODUCTION

A keto or ketogenic diet is a low-carb, moderate protein, a higher-fat eating routine that can help you consume fat all the more viably. It has numerous advantages for weight reduction, wellbeing, and execution, as appeared in more than 50 studies.1 That's the reason it's suggested by a developing number of specialists and medical care practitioners.2

A keto diet is particularly helpful for losing overabundance muscle to fat ratio, decreasing craving, and improving sort 2 diabetes or metabolic syndrome.34

Here, you'll sort out some way to eat a keto diet subject to authentic sustenance. Begin with our visual aids, plans, supper plans, and basic 2-week Get Started program. Its start and end you need to persuade keto.

WHAT IS THE KETO DIET?

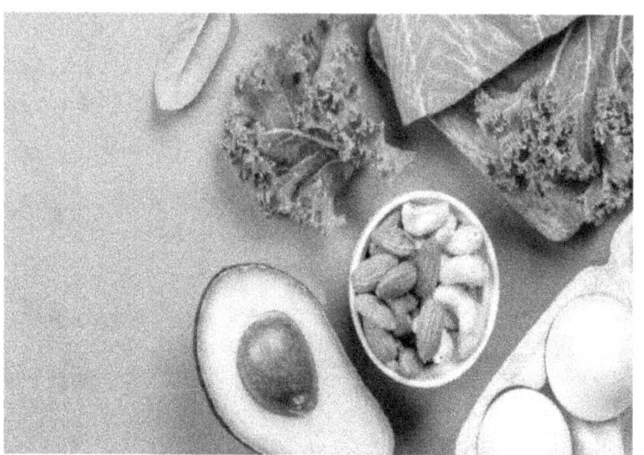

You may have heard the old low-fat weight-reduction mantra, "Fat makes you fat." It's really not excessively straightforward. Your cerebrum and body profit by solid fats, paying little heed to what diet you follow. Eating keto implies eating more fats and fewer carbs, which changes the manner in which your body transforms food into energy.

Think about your body as a crossbreed vehicle. You're worked to depend on starches, similar to bread and pasta, for fuel. Your digestion is intended to transform carbs into glucose for energy. However, much the same as a half breed can run on gas or power, your body has another approach to make energy: fat.

In the event that you eat not many carbs, more fat, and moderate protein, your body enters ketosis: a metabolic state where you consume fat rather than carbs for fuel.[1]

In ketosis, your body produces ketones, an elective wellspring of fuel. Ketones are liable for a great deal of the keto benefits you may have caught wind of, as fewer desires, more mental ability, and enduring energy.

The keto diet is one way to deal with get your body to make ketones. Your body can likewise create ketones when you're discontinuous fasting or taking keto supplements like Bulletproof Brain Octane C8 MCT Oil, otherwise known as the most ketogenic MCT oil.

KETO DIET BENEFITS

Ketosis conveys a lot of medical advantages other than consuming fat. Your digestion works contrastingly on keto, and individuals report the accompanying adjustments in their perspective and body.

EXPANDED ENERGY

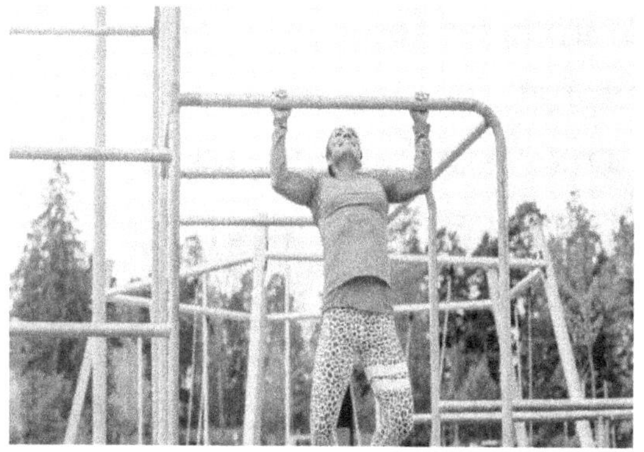

Over 60% of your psyche is fat, so it needs a predictable store of fat to keep the engine humming.[2] The quality fats you eat on a ketogenic diet accomplish more than feeding your everyday exercises—they likewise feed your cerebrum.

At the point when your body utilizes ketones for fuel, you won't encounter a similar energy crashes or mind haze as you do when you're eating a lot of carbs. You know the inclination you get subsequent to having a major bowl of pasta for lunch? Your glucose levels crash in the wake of preparing each one of those carbs and the remainder of the day becomes nap time.

That is not the situation on the keto diet. In metabolic fat-consuming mode, your body can take advantage of fat stores for energy. Ketosis additionally assists the mind with making mitochondria, the force generators in your cells.[3] More energy in your cells implies more energy to complete stuff.

FEWER CRAVINGS

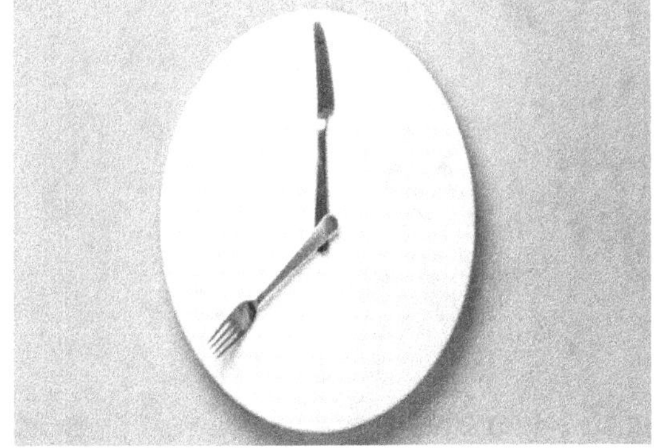

Ketones stifle ghrelin, your craving hormone. They additionally increment cholecystokinin (CCK), which causes you to feel full.[4] Reduced hunger implies it's simpler to go for longer periods without eating, which urges your body to plunge into its fat stores for energy.

Fat is a satisfying macronutrient, which implies it causes you feel more full, longer.[5] On a high-fat eating routine, you'll invest less energy nibbling and additional time handling your daily agenda.

Related: Learn how Bulletproof MCT Oil fulfills hunger.

WEIGHT MANAGEMENT

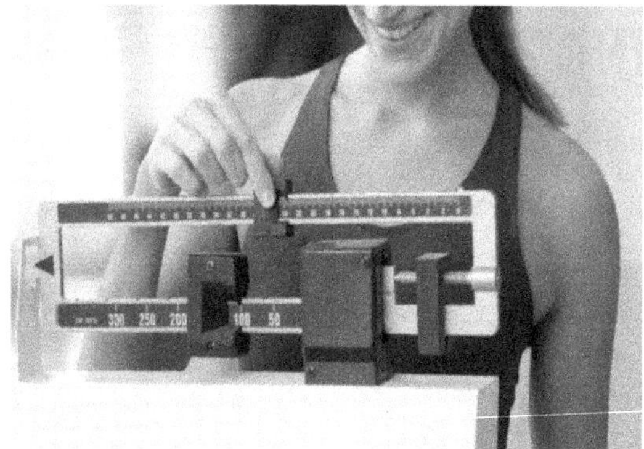

A few people utilize the keto diet to remain at a sound weight. In contrast to glucose, ketones can't be put away as fat since they aren't used in a similar way. This may appear to be nonsensical in the event that you partner keto with heaps of bacon and cheddar. Yet, truly, the keto diet can uphold weight the executives by consuming fat and control longings.

DECREASED INFLAMMATION

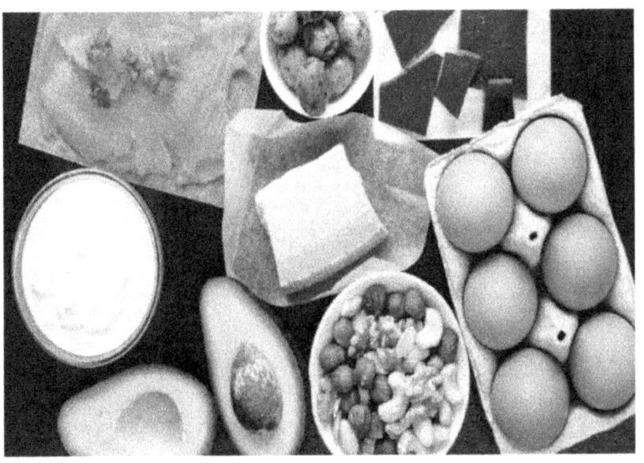

Aggravation is your body's normal reaction to an intruder it considers unsafe. An excessive amount of aggravation is awful news since it builds your danger of medical issues. A keto diet can lessen aggravation in the body by turning off incendiary pathways and creating less free extremists contrasted with glucose.

KINDS OF KETO DIETS

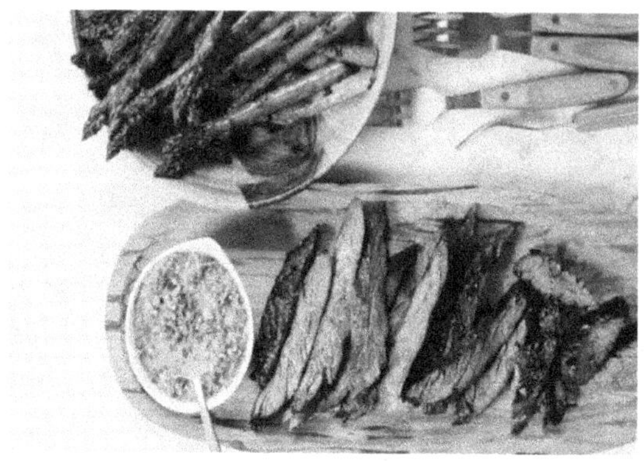

The keto diet for tenderfoots seems like all fat, no carbs, and bunches of bacon and cheddar—yet that is not the situation. There are various ways to deal with this way of eating, and it's alright to test to discover what works for you. A few people do well with somewhat more carbs in their weight control plans, and that is entirely alright. Here are a couple of various ways to deal with a high-fat, low-carb diet:

- **Standard keto**: This is regularly 75% fat, 20% protein, and 5% net carbs a day, consistently. Some keto adherents eat as not many as 20 grams of net carbs every day.

- **Cyclical keto**: You adhere to a standard keto diet a large portion of the week. One to two days every week, you have a "carb refeed" in which you eat somewhat more carbs. For instance, you may eat roughly 150 grams of net carbs during carb refeed days.

- **Directed keto**: You notice the standard keto diet, yet eat more carbs 30 minutes to an hour around works out. The glucose is intended to support the execution and your re-visitation of ketosis after the exercise. In the event that your energy is enduring in the rec center during keto, this way of eating may work for you.

- **Dirty keto**: Dirty keto follows a similar proportion of dietary fats, proteins, and carbs as the normal keto diet, yet with a turn: It doesn't make a difference where those macronutrients come from.

- **Moderate keto**: Eat high fat with roughly 100-150 grams of net carbs every day. Individuals who experience issues with different types of keto once in a while improve this eating routine on the grounds that confining carbs can at times meddle with hormonal capacity and energy levels.

THE MOST EFFECTIVE METHOD TO BEGIN THE KETO DIET

Try not to dump the carbs at the same time. Continue perusing to figure out how to see whether the keto way of life is ideal for you.

START SLOWLY AND MINDFULLY

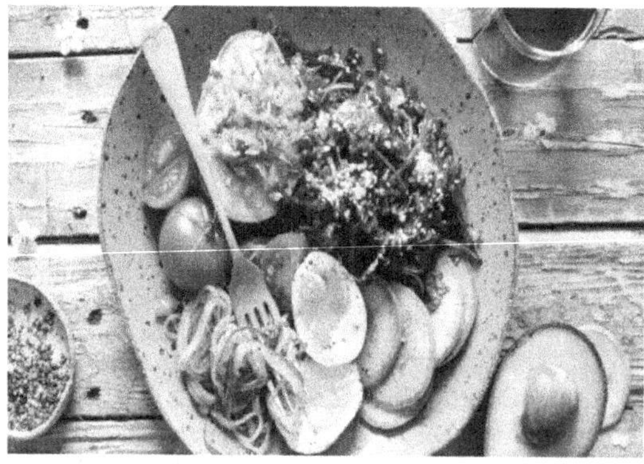

To get the best thought of which style of keto works for you, attempt an alternate style of keto for at any rate a month.

Make it simple on yourself by following your carbs, fat, and protein utilizing a food following application like MyFitnessPal and My Macros+. This will make it simple to set objectives dependent on fat and carb consumption as opposed to stressing over calories. Eat until you're full, and tune in to your body.

In particular, check in with your body as you go. Is it true that you are most honed with a week by week carb refeed, or improve on a full ketogenic diet? Do you wear out when you plunge under 100 grams of carbs every day?

There's a ton of variety inside lower-carb diets, and a few people feel their best with various styles of eating. Locate a decent equilibrium that turns out best for your body.

EAT QUALITY FATS AND MODERATE PROTEIN

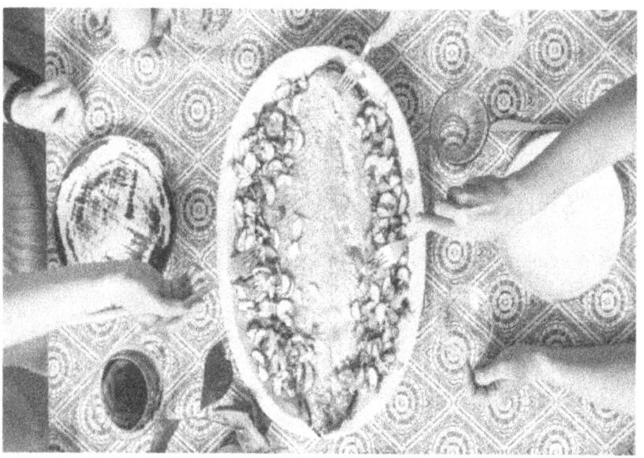

Dissimilar to the Atkins Diet, which is high in protein, a keto diet tries not to eat an excessive amount of protein. This is on the grounds that a lot of protein can transform into glucose in a cycle called gluconeogenesis, which removes you from ketosis.

There's somewhat of an expectation to absorb information when you're discovering what to eat on keto. Extensively, it's ideal to get your dietary fat from supplement thick, entire food sources. That implies eating more nourishments like avocados, coconut oil, olive oil, and margarine (or Bulletproof Grass-Fed Ghee). Your protein admission should principally come from greasy cuts of protein like salmon and, indeed, bacon.

THE MOST EFFECTIVE METHOD TO KNOW WHEN YOU'RE IN KETOSIS

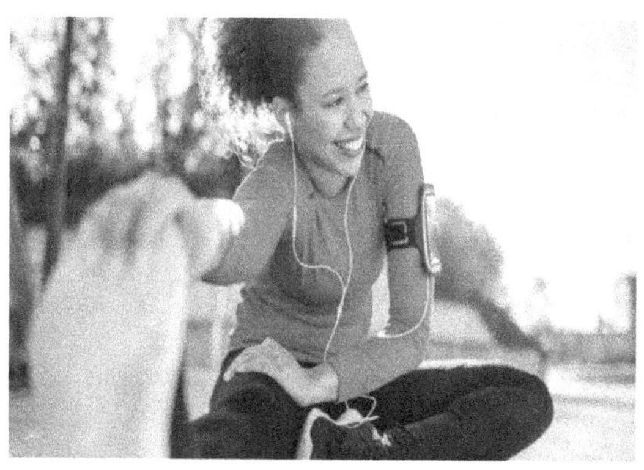

What measure of time does it need to get into ketosis? It can take somewhere in the range of 2-3 days to half a month to enter ketosis, contingent upon your body's capacity to adjust to consuming fat for fuel.

As your body changes, it's entirely expected to experience the keto influenza during the main week or thereabouts. You may encounter side effects like cerebrum haze, muscle throbs, and even a surprising intuition regarding your mouth (otherwise known as "keto breath").

When you enter ketosis, you'll notice changes like fewer yearnings, clear-headedness, and expanded energy. Contingent upon how your body acclimates to this way of eating, you may likewise see keto results. In case you're experiencing difficulty resting or managing low energy, you may feel better with marginally more carbs in your eating regimen. Analysis with carb cycling to discover what works for you.

KETO RECIPES.

You can even now appreciate tasty, low-carb nourishments you'll anticipate eating as a feature of your keto feast plan. There are even keto-accommodating renditions of your most loved carb-weighty nourishments, similar to hotcakes and treats.

Here are a couple of our number one low-carb plans. Peruse Bulletproof Recipes to discover more keto-accommodating dinner thoughts.

Impenetrable Coffee

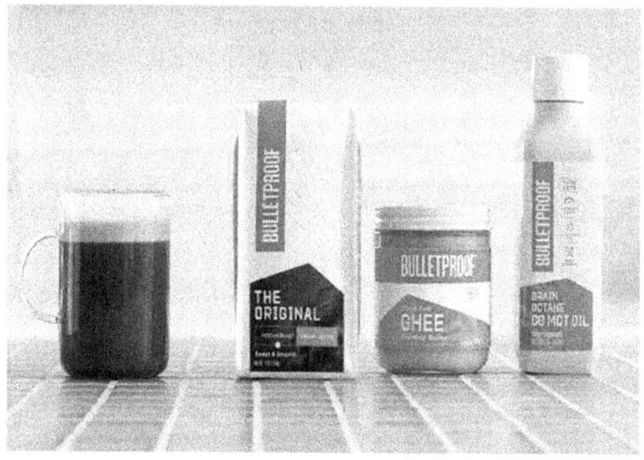

Start your day with quality fats that keep you going solid throughout the morning. To prepare this keto espresso formula, you'll mix grass-took care of spread or Grass-Fed Ghee with affirmed clean Bulletproof espresso beans and Brain Octane C8 MCT Oil to make a smooth, foamy latte that will keep you stimulated and fulfilled.

Keto Coconut Flour Pancakes

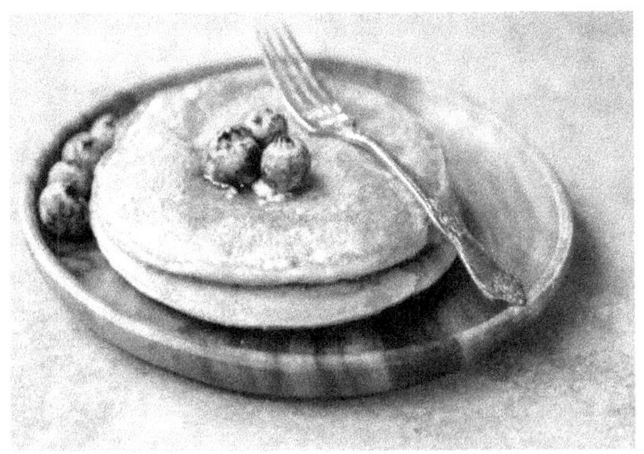

Indeed, you can at present appreciate hotcakes on a low-carb diet. This simple keto formula utilizes coconut flour, vanilla, and Grass-Fed Ghee to convey flavorful flapjacks at simply 2.2 net carbs per cake.

This simple burger plate of mixed greens highlights avocado, caramelized onions, and a tasty aioli. Have all the fulfillment of a burger with under 7 grams of net carbs. The solitary distinction is you're exchanging the bun for a bowl.

Eating your veggies never tasted this great. Verdant greens are finished off with eggs and smoked salmon to make a delightful, supplement thick serving of mixed greens that fulfills your macros and your tastebuds. The dressing is made with Brain Octane C8 MCT Oil, which is a flavorless method to help ketone production

Lemon Drizzle Cake

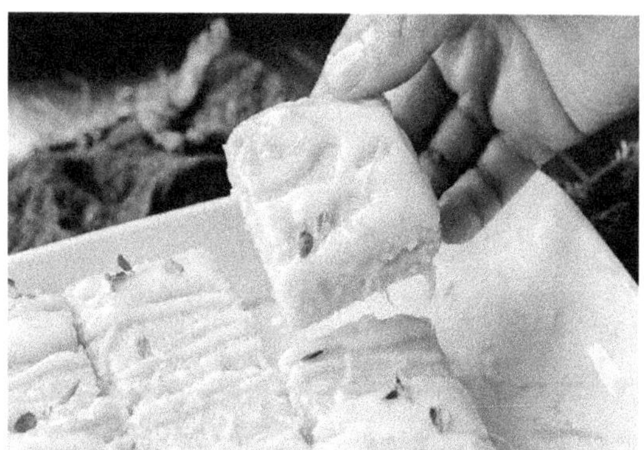

Get the flavor of summer any season with this simple Lemon Drizzle Cake, in addition to protein support from Bulletproof Collagen Protein powder. One cut is about 9.5 grams of net carbs. Use keto-accommodating fluid sugar rather than maple syrup for a much more keto-accommodating cut.